MOVEMENT THAT MATTERS

A PRACTICAL APPROACH TO DEVELOPING OPTIMAL FUNCTIONAL MOVEMENT SKILLS

Paul Chek

**Illustrations
Charlie Aligaen**

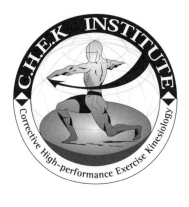

A C.H.E.K Institute Publication

For information contact:
C.H.E.K INSTITUTE
609 South Vulcan Avenue, Suite 101, Encinitas, CA 92024, USA
Ph: 1.800.552.8789 or 760.632.6360
Fax: 760.632.1037
E-mail: ginfo@chekinstitute.com
Web page: www.chekinstitute.com

ISBN 1-58387-002-4
Chek, Paul W.
Illustrator: Charlie Aligaen
Editors: Cara Burke
        Bryan Walsh
        Christina Walsh
Book and Cover Design: Charlie Aligaen, Cara Burke and Penthea Crozier

Contents

Teaching movement and developing motor skills in rehabilitation and/or personal training clientele can be accomplished simply and effectively! Today, the exercise and rehabilitation professional faces many challenges with regard to exercise prescription and program design. These challenges include time pressures, confusion about treatment philosophy, and information overload. Due to the emergence of an ever-increasing number of experts, coupled with the easy accessibility of the Internet, practitioners are faced with a large number of seemingly convincing, but frequently conflicting, opinions from leaders in their fields. Information overload has become a reality, resulting in *paralysis by analysis* among many professionals. The academic literature is frequently the expression of an isolationist mentality. You may find the information frustrating and relatively useless.

This book ties together current research and clinical observations with valuable knowledge from the past. Much of the valuable information from the past has been inundated by "modern" information and forgotten. The information contained here will provide the exercise and rehabilitation professional with an effective approach to assessing movement skills and improving function in their clients.

WHAT IS FUNCTIONAL MOVEMENT?

Func.tion.al 1. capable of operating or functioning 2. having or serving a utilitarian purpose; capable of serving the purpose for which it was designed.

(Webster's Encyclopedic Unabridged Dictionary of the English Language, 2nd Edition, 1996)

The word "functional" is commonly used to indicate "useful," "applicable" or something that works. Today there are trainers and gym programs, therapists and rehabilitation clinics, chiropractors and doctors all claiming to provide or prescribe "functional exercise." Are these programs actually living up to the meaning of the term "functional" with regard to exercise prescription, or are they riding yet another fad? Below are the guidelines used for prescribing "functional exercise" at the C.H.E.K Institute (Table 1). To determine if an exercise is truly functional, compare it to the following table; in most cases it must meet all six characteristics to be considered functional.

Characteristics of Functional Exercise

1. Comparable reflex profile (Righting and Equilibrium reflexes)
2. Maintenance of your center of gravity over your own base of support
   ✓ Static postural component
   ✓ Dynamic postural component
3. Generalized motor program compatibility
4. Open/closed chain compatibility
5. Relevant biomotor abilities
6. Isolation to integration

Table 1

1. REFLEX PROFILE

As upright human beings, we must move across the earth under the influence of gravity. On a day-to-day basis, we do everything from climbing mountains to working at construction sites and factories to riding subway trains, buses, motorcycles and skateboards. Each activity we do requires activation of specialized reflexes intended to protect us from hurting ourselves. These reflexes provide us with such abilities as putting our hands out to regain our balance after a bus begins driving before we have had a chance to get seated.

These reflex reactions are commonly broken into two major groups:

- ✓ Righting reactions
- ✓ Equilibrium reactions

The majority of our righting and tilting responses should be built into the nervous system before age three.[1]

Righting reactions can be broken into five different reflexes that serve the following functions: keeping the head in a normal position, righting the body to a normal position and adjusting the body parts in relation to the head and vice versa.[1] These reactions are called:

a. Labyrinthine-righting reflexes acting on the head
b. Body-righting reflexes acting on the head
c. Neck-righting reflexes
d. Body-righting reflexes acting on the body
e. Optical-righting reflexes

Labyrinthine-righting reflexes
Stimulation of the proprioceptors of the labyrinth causes changes in tone of the neck muscles which brings the head into its natural position in space.

Body-righting reflexes
Reflexive effects of the neck muscles which bring the head into the correct position in space caused by stimulation of pressoreceptors in the body wall by contact with the ground.

Neck-righting reflexes
Changes in position of the head cause alterations in tone of the neck muscles through stimulation of proprioceptors in the labyrinth which bring the head into its correct position in space; stimulation of proprioceptors in the neck muscles in turn causes reflex movements of the limbs which bring the body into the normal position in relation to the head.

Table 2

In addition to righting reactions, we have equilibrium reactions. These reactions are developed in us as children for the purpose of maintaining or regaining control over the body's center of gravity, thus preventing us from falling. According to Barnes, there are several categories of equilibrium reactions:[2]

    a. Protective reaction of the arms and legs
    b. Tilting reactions
    c. Postural fixating reactions

Although there are many work and sport activities that require both righting and equilibrium reactions, there are numerous activities that require predominantly either one or the other.

   ✓ Righting reactions tend to be dominant when moving across a fixed or stable surface, such as a sidewalk, or even a balance beam in gymnastics.

   ✓ Equilibrium or tilting reactions are more dominant when the supportive surface moves underneath us. Wind surfing, working on a fishing boat in the open sea, riding a horse, a motorcycle or a subway train are examples of activities using righting and equilibrium reactions together, but may require a dominance of equilibrium reactions.[3]

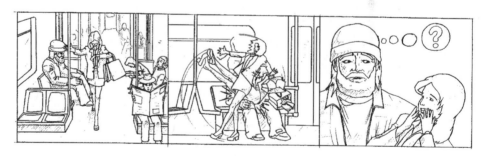

Figure 1

Consider riding a subway train. If you are not holding onto the pole in the subway car when it takes off and you have slow tilting reflexes, you can imagine what will happen! (Figure 1) The same could be said of any activity that requires a reflex response to maintain an upright posture or protect the body. Vladimir Janda stated that if we could speed the reflex response time of our bodies by 50%, we would reduce the chances of acquiring an orthopedic injury by about 80%.[4]

Application: When selecting exercises for your patient or client, it is important to identify the dominant reflex profile in the activity for which they are conditioning. In sports such as equestrian, surfing or motorcycle racing, it is very important to determine which aspect of the task is most challenging to your client.

Case History 1: A motocross racer has a difficult time sliding through corners, but can handle straight-away riding and jumping.

Solution: This individual would likely benefit from exercises that emphasize the tilting aspect of an equilibrium response. One such exercise is kneeling on a Swiss Ball and catching a medicine ball tossed from the side (Figure 2). This would aid in improving the rider's ability to respond more quickly to the motorcycle when sliding through corners.

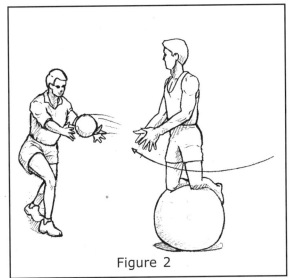
Figure 2

Case History 2: Another motocross racer is competent in the corners, but has a difficult time controlling the bike through rough sections of the course due to a lack of strength or strength endurance (Figure 3-A).

Solution: A circuit emphasizing righting responses and consisting of a series of exercises organized in a sequence of descending neurological demand would be useful in this scenario. For example, a bent-over row kneeling on the Swiss Ball (Figure 3-B), followed by single-leg stance exercises

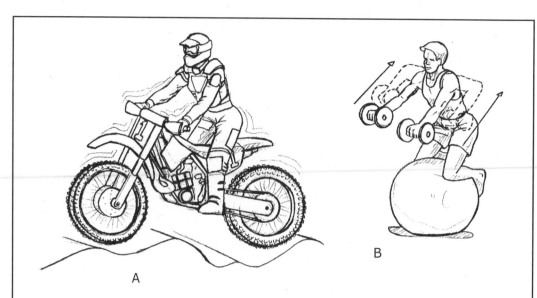

Figure 3A & B

The racer must maintain his center of gravity over his base of support, which is unstable during a motocross race and continues to be unstable during the Swiss Ball kneeling bent-over row (B). Although righting and equilibrium responses are activated in the body at the same time, for a motocross racer, this exercise will be much less challenging to the equilibrium response than the exercise in Figure 2, particularly with an equal load in each hand and movement predominantly in the sagittal plane, just as during straight-away riding. Should movement of the ball impede his ability to perform the exercise, placing the ball on a soft mat will slow the ball, allowing greater use of a righting response and allowing him to place more emphasis in the plane of his comparable sport-specific weakness.

and finishing with two-legged stance exercises would be beneficial to this athlete. The next progression would be to do single-arm-opposite-leg cable pushing, followed by single arm abductions with a dumbbell (standing on the same leg), alternating between left and right sides for equal repetitions and finally finishing with a bout of Bodyblade® work. The intensive interval method (~ 30 seconds per exercise) would be optimal. After 1:00 minute of rest, the circuit would be repeated up to 5–10 times, depending on the condition of the motocross racer. The key factor in selecting work volume is to make sure bad motor skills are not being developed or reinforced by fatigue, as this may have a negative effect on racing performance.

Using a protocol such as one of those described above will also serve to enhance postural fixating reactions. This is important for the maintenance and development of any client's or patient's reflex profile, as well as sound motor engram development (expanded upon below).

2. MAINTENANCE OF CENTER OF GRAVITY OVER BASE OF SUPPORT

In most activities of daily life (aside from sitting in a chair, driving a car or using most of the "non-functional" machines littering the gyms worldwide), we must maintain our center of gravity over our own base of support. Maintaining center of gravity over base of support (balance) is so vitally important that, under normal circumstances, we master it within the first 24 months of our life.

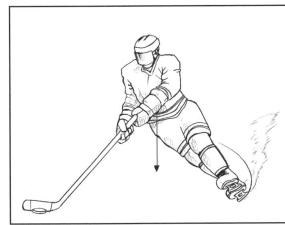

Figure 4
While turning, the hockey player's center of gravity is well outside of his base of support. He is supported by his inertial energy and his connection to the ice by his sharp skate blades. Should he lose footing or be stopped abruptly, you can clearly see that he would fall over unless he repositioned one leg under his center of gravity (indicated by arrow).

When our center of gravity goes outside our base of support, we are more likely to fall over. The only exceptions are cases where our own inertial energy will hold us up, such as with an ice hockey player turning quickly (Figure 4) or when we are being supported by an outside force, such as the wind while riding a sail board (Figure 5). In functional situations such as those demonstrated in Figures 4 and 5, we must draw heavily on our body's ability to integrate muscle groups and on our righting and tilting responses.

If you consider a typical daily activity such as putting a suitcase in the trunk of one's car (Figure 6), it becomes obvious that our nervous system must be capable of integrating both static and dynamic postural functions.[5] To better appreciate these terms, let's explore them individually.

Static postural stability

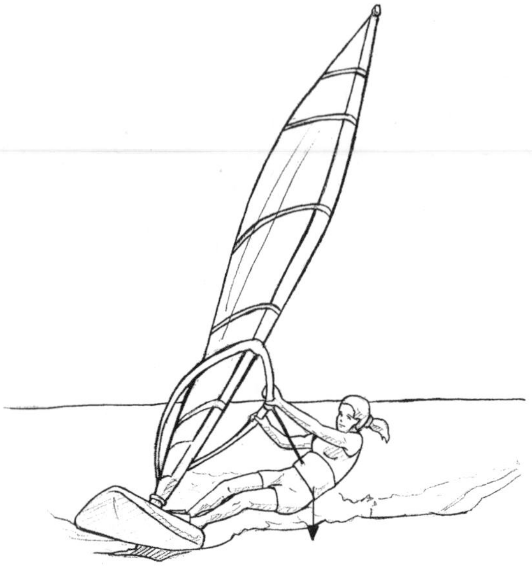

While standing upright, the force of gravity will actually serve to assist in stabilization of a well-aligned body. Most of us know people who cannot stand still for a period of time without feeling pressure in their neck or back. This often leads them to auto-manipulate, or adjust their own spine, in an attempt to decrease activation of mechanoreceptors in ligaments and joint capsules surrounding the subluxed joints.

When we lean forward in a field of gravity, there is what is termed a *flexion moment* placed on our body. Leaning backward or behind the mid-frontal plane produces an *extension moment*. As we lean progressively further forward, the moment increases because more of our body weight is forward of the axis of rotation. However, the flexion moment is not exponential with regard to degrees of forward lean. It rises quickly during the first 30° of forward bending, at which point the rate of increase slows.[6] The moment is almost the same at 30° of forward bend as it is at 45°.

The larger the flexion moment, the harder our extensor muscles have to work to keep us from falling over. When

Figure 5
The windsurfer uses the force of the wind and support of the boom to maintain a body position in which her center of gravity (see arrow) is significantly displaced from her base of support. Should the wind suddenly stop, she would be unable to maintain her balance due to the lateral displacement of her center of gravity. Maintenance of her position while windsurfing requires constant integration of her body segments with the action of the sail and board. This requires constant activation and utilization of all aspects of righting and equilibrium responses.

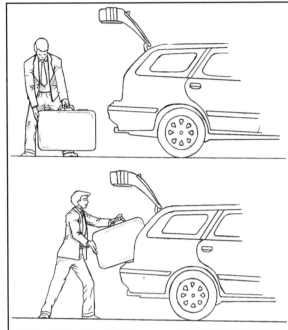

Figure 6
While bending over to pick up a suitcase or any weighted object, the erectors of the back and hips must activate to support the trunk as a working platform (static stability). The concept of stability can be seen during such activities as putting on make-up or brushing teeth, where the torso is held in a specific position against gravity. Dynamic stability, as seen here, relates to the fact that as the suitcase is transferred into the car, the joints must be dynamically controlled so that joint health is maintained and the body is not injured. When the stabilizer mechanisms of the body work correctly, an optimal axis of rotation is always maintained within each joint complex.

holding an object in our hands, such as the suitcase shown in Figure 6, the flexion moment rises in proportion to the weight being held. Therefore, the work that must be done by our body to keep us upright also increases. To appreciate the concept of static stability, consider how tired your back can get while simply leaning forward over a sink to brush your teeth. Then add the weight of a suitcase and the additional load created by the lever arm of your trunk and arms and it becomes clear why people hurt their backs while on vacation or while performing daily activities.

Static stability is the ability to hold our body in any position that allows us to carry out a goal or task against the load of our extremity(ies), trunk and any other additional load handled by our body. In Figure 6, the person putting the suitcase in the car must have adequate static stability to hold himself up in a field of gravity. Failure to have adequate static stability in the muscular system will result in pathological loading of ligaments. This is a common source of joint instability, particularly in the lumbar spine.

Dynamic stability: The ability to maintain an optimal instantaneous axis of rotation in any joint or combination of joints in any space/time combination.

To better understand the concept of dynamic stability, let us continue to use Figure 6 as an example. Static stability provides the working platform from which the suitcase could be picked up and moved from the ground into the trunk. Dynamic stability requires that each joint complex in the body be stabilized by its respective stabilizer muscles in such a way that it functions within the parameters necessary to maintain optimal joint health. For example, from the forward bend position (static stability), the arms primarily change the location of the suitcase (relative to the body) and handle the load dynamically. The rotator cuff and the large muscles around the shoulder must be intelligently timed to make sure the shoulder joint does not get damaged by the load; the same principle applies to all parts of the body involved in the dynamic transport of the load.

When the joint stabilizers are healthy, the joint will maintain a concentric axis of rotation. There are exceptions to this rule, such as in a joint complex with multiple axes of rotation. For the purpose of explanation, I will keep it simple and stick to the concept of maintaining an optimal axis of rotation. A concentric axis of rotation results in a joint rotating toward or around its optimal *instantaneous axis of rotation* (Figure 7A). This constitutes *good dynamic stability*. If a joint com-

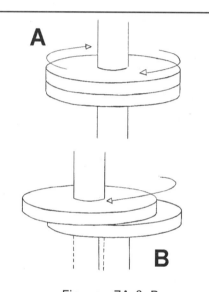

Figures 7A & B
Optimal Instantaneous Axis of Rotation: A. While maintaining a concentric axis, the two joint surfaces will not move away from each other under influence of a rotational force. B. When stabilizer and/or joint function is aberrant, an eccentric axis of rotation may exist, during which joint surfaces move away from each other. An eccentric axis of motion is commonly associated with ligamentous stress and joint derangement.

plex is not stabilized properly, any load, be it intrinsic or extrinsic, will impart an eccentric rotation to the joint complex. An eccentric rotation is one in which the joint surfaces move away from an optimal instantaneous axis of rotation, producing an eccentric axis of rotation (Figure 7B). An eccentric rotation of any joint complex, particularly under load, may produce what is commonly referred to by chiropractors as a *subluxation*.

Luxation: a dislocation of a joint

Application: To develop functional strength with a high level of carry-over to work, sport or recreation, we must apply the principles of static and dynamic stability through optimal selection of exercises. It should be immediately apparent that if we use a machine that supports our body in any way (particularly seated, prone, supine or leaning), we are not activating the body's static stabilizer or postural system. This is a critical concept to grasp when one considers the harsh reality that *stability must always precede force generation.* As the old saying goes, "You can't fire a cannon from a canoe!" This is exactly why you may see a noticeable difference between your performance during a Smith squat and a free squat, or even more dramatically, the difference between leg press performance versus squat or deadlift performance.

Intrinsic Stabilizers:
muscles crossing any given joint complex

Extrinsic Stabilizers:
muscles crossing multiple working joints

To further clarify the difference between machines and functional exercise, consider the following. Any time a machine guides the load using a fixed, or even semi-fixed, axis of motion, there is a reduction in the need to recruit the body's own intrinsic and extrinsic stabilizers. An example of dynamic stabilization is seen when a novice lifter is introduced to an exercise as simple as a dumbbell bench press. Often the dumbbells look like they have a mind of their own for the first several training sessions. Take the dumbbells out of the hands of that same client and walk the person over to any chest press machine and they will perform as though they were born in a gym.

Quite frankly, it really does not matter how strong anyone is on a machine exercise. To go one step further (this may upset some meatheads), there is a VERY POOR correlation between strength during any supported lift (such as a bench press, prone row, Smith squat or split squat) and any functional lift or task such as breaking through the line in football, controlling an opponent in wrestling or making it through a slalom course in water or on snow.

There are several reasons for this:

✓   Stability always limits performance. As far as the body is concerned, the health of the working joints is of greater importance than your desire to move an object. To ensure joint, tendon and muscle safety, the body has a nicely developed system of neuromuscular and neuromechanical receptors located throughout muscles, tendons and joints. These range from spindle cells in muscles to the type I, II, III and IV mechanoreceptors in the joint capsule and Golgi tendon organs in the tendons.[7] If the exercises used in the training environment do not adequately prepare the static and dynamic stabilizer systems, faulty and/or pathological joint motion during standing functional exercises is almost inevitable.

✓   If the body perceives that the compression, torsion, sheer and/or stretch forces acting on any working joint complex are a threat to the survival of the system, it produces an inhibitory response, or down-regulation of the motor neurons feeding the muscles crossing the jeopardized joint structure(s). This response is well documented in orthopedic literature and has been clinically proven countless times; injection of as little as 50 cc's of fluid into the knee joint or swelling within the shoulder joint results in significant loss of strength due to stretching of relevant mechanorceptors, producing inhibition of the muscles.

✓ With very few exceptions, exercises performed in an environment that provides stability to the body do not require integration of the upper and lower extremities. This is a critical concept to grasp as the brain develops functional force in the neuromusculoskeletal system by commanding movements, not muscles.

An additional, and very real, consideration is that the torso, or core musculature, not only provides the initiation of stabilization for the extremities, but also serves to transfer force from the legs to the arms and vice versa.[8] A very effective, and often emotional experience for the "Big Bencher" comes when simply comparing their bench press performance to their standing cable push performance (Figure 8A & B). Having performed this very test on many amateur and professional athletes, I can tell you it is rare to find an athlete who can perform a standing push with a split stance using more than 30% of their maximum bench press or a single-leg standing push with more than 5% of their maximum bench press. This is an important point when you consider that in nearly all sports,

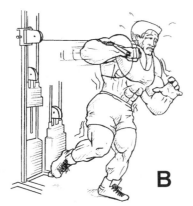

Figures 8A & B
A. Classically, an athlete who spends all their time developing a "big bench" will lack integrative training or ability.
B. Most of the "big benchers," or even "little benchers" who train with isolation techniques, perform very poorly during the Standing Single Leg Cable Push Test.

force is commonly applied while predominantly standing on one leg or the other! Those who have performed well during the standing cable push tests have generally had a background in Olympic lifting, martial arts, wrestling, dance or other functional exercise systems, or surprisingly, no specific training at all. The athletes exhibiting the greatest difficulty have been those exposed to bodybuilding (isolation) training; the longer they have trained with isolation techniques, the more poorly they perform in general.

    ✓   Motor patterns developed by supported exercises do not carry over well to standing exercises. This is expanded upon below.

By now you may be wondering how to apply this information. Simply follow these guidelines.

1. Choose exercises that have a high correlation to the functional demands of your client's or patient's work or sport environment.

2. Place these exercises before non-functional exercises during a workout due to high neurological demand. Also, exercise form degenerates quickly when functional exercises are attempted after the body is fatigued from other exercises. There are only two exceptions in which non-functional exercises may come first:

> 1. When conditioning an elite athlete who is experienced at weight training, exibits functional stability at optimal training intensities and needs to have their nervous system challenged
>
> 2. During a base conditioning program where mass is of greater concern than neuromuscular integration training. For example, a football player lacking chest and shoulder mass may perform the bench press prior to squating to allow optimal enery and intensity for the primary objective – a stronger chest and shoulders. In this case, simply remember this rule, "if you are going to isolate, you must then integrate!"[9]

With any exercise that does not require us to maintain our center of gravity over our own base of support, we are not learning the necessary *skill* to apply force while controlling our own center of gravity. This is one of the reasons that many of the "big guys" on teams get severely out-performed by "little guys!"

SKILL vs. ABILITY

Skill: Consists of the ability to bring about some end result with maximum certainty and minimum outlay of energy, or of time and energy.[10]

Ability: Genetically determined and largely unmodified by practice or experience. Abilities can therefore be thought of as the basic "equipment" that people are born with.[10]

Physical Ability: Refers to one's current orthopedic status. For example, to perform a full squat or lunge, you must have the *ability* to move your hip joints through normal ranges of flexion and extension.

---

3. GENERALIZED MOTOR PROGRAM COMPATIBILITY

There are hundreds of exercises and almost as many movement philosophies that can be used to teach your client how to move, each backed by one or more credible experts. So which do you use? The concept of generalized motor programs as a means of storing movement patterns was propounded by Schmidt.[10] One of the primary reasons motor learning experts have explored the concept of the generalized motor program is because many believe the brain does not have adequate storage capacity to hold the myriad of programs one could generate throughout a lifetime of movement. Schmidt has proposed that the brain stores *generalized motor programs*. Each motor program can be used for groups of movements that have the same relative timing.

A typical example of a generalized motor program is easily found in the squat movement pattern. Research shows that there is a very poor carryover from isolation exercises (such as knee extensions, hamstring curls and the leg press) to improving one's vertical jump. At the same time, there is

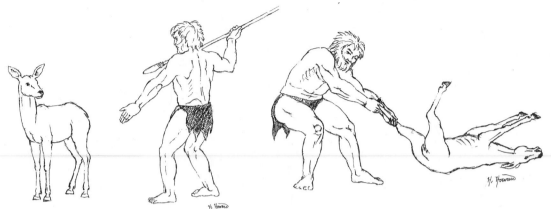

Figure 9: Twist Pattern

Figure 10: Pull Pattern

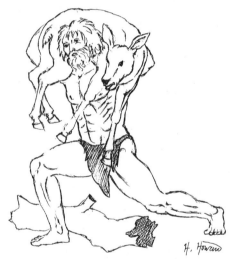

Figure 11: Lunge Pattern

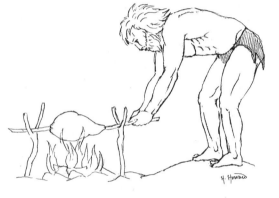

Figure 12: Bend Pattern

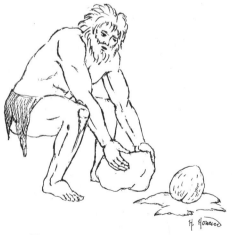

Figure 13: Squat Pattern

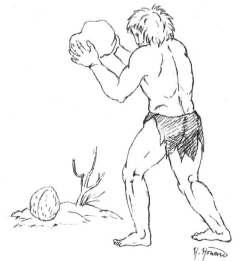

Figure 14: Push Pattern

research finding that resisted squat training provides significant improvement in vertical jump performance. This coincides with Schmidt's theory of the generalized motor program, as the squat and the jump use a similar movement pattern. The same could be said for the power clean and the vertical jump.

Prior to finding Schmidt's research, I was having great success in the rehabilitation of my orthopedic patients using a system I developed, the *Primal Pattern*™ *System*. I hypothesized that the selective pressures of evolution must have resulted in a human anatomy that was specifically designed to meet the demands made by nature. I also proposed that if one could not twist, pull, lunge, bend, squat and push from the standing position or could not effectively ambulate (gait), then chances of survival would dwindle severely (Figures 9–15).[11]

Today, we are nothing more than cavemen with fancy clothes, sitting at desks. As I have seen numerous times in my practice, when someone cannot efficiently perform any of the *Primal Pattern* movements at a level of subconscious competency, there are almost always injuries lurking, if not already present. To effectively teach our clients how to move, we must determine which *Primal Patterns* are most commonly used in their work and/or sports environment and assess their ability to perform these patterns.

Application: Based on my clinical experience and research, functional exercises assist in developing *functional movement skills* when they closely resemble a movement pattern that is commonly used in the client's work or sports environment. The further one deviates from a pattern that has the same, or similar general characteristics or *relative timing,* the less likely the exercise is to be useful!

To determine where to focus your efforts in a rehabilitation or conditioning program, you must assess your client's ability to perform the *Primal Pattern* movements in their pure form. This generally means testing the client with loads and implements that are relevant to the activities they perform.

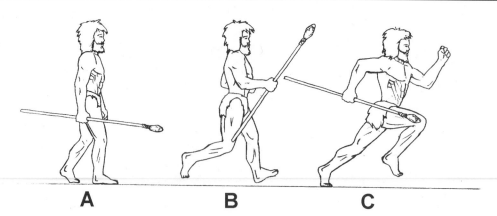

Figures 15A – C

As primal beings, we had to transport ourselves predominantly by gait. Research implies that we use different motor patterns at different speeds of gait, with the most likely shift in relative timing of generalized motor patterns coming at the transition from (A) walking, to (B) running and finally (C) all out sprinting.[26] It is suggested that the shift from the more efficient walking pattern to the running or sprint patterns may be related to conservation of energy, which was critical during our developmental years.[22]

For example, one would not obtain good results with a female secretary who roller-blades for exercise by loading her with 4 RM (Repitition Maximum) in the lunge!

Using the example of the secretary above, you could ask her to simply perform a lunge at body-weight intensity and analyze her performance. If you know she has a child ranging from newborn to age 3, chances are good she carries the child frequently while performing house chores. With this knowledge at hand, your most realistic test result may come from asking her to perform the squat pattern while holding a medicine ball, weighing approximately the same as her child, to her chest.

To keep your testing procedures within the scope of reality for this particular woman, you may then ask her to drop the ball on the floor in preparation for the bend test. Ask her to pick up the ball, watching carefully to see how she performs in the bend pattern. Her brain may perceive the load as significant enough to opt for the squat pattern to lift the ball, which is valuable information with regard to her ability to assess and solve physical challenges. Frequently, people are injured or at risk of injury because they do not have the motor skills or problem-solving skills to make intelligent decisions about which pattern to use for a given task or how to best position their body to accept and transfer a load. The ability to perform such tasks with good form is an indicator of *movement skill.*

ASSESSING COMPOUND MOVEMENTS

Another reality is that the body effectively compounds *Primal Pattern* movements to create other more complex movements. This is particularly the case with single-arm pushing, single-arm pulling, and twisting actions performed from the standing position (Figure 8B). A very simple and common example of this can be both seen and experienced by either watching someone throw a ball, or throwing the ball yourself (Figure 16). To propel the object, the body performs a lunge, followed by a twist, and summates the forces of these movements with a push in the form of medial shoulder rotation, elbow extension and accessory movements at the wrist and hand (Figures 17A–C).

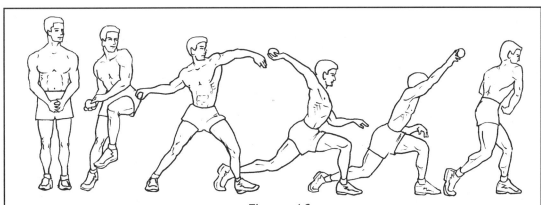

Figure 16

To the untrained eye, throwing a ball looks like one indivisible movement or *motor pattern.* In reality, throwing or pitching a ball may be three motor patterns, which are likely to have been learned in *chunks* as smaller motor programs (Figures 17A–C). Once learned, the motor pattern will be stored in one's long-term memory and accessed with the cognitive command "throw the ball."

The concept of the generalized motor program explains why so many forms of exercise simply do not improve function or serve as optimal injury prevention. Someone who subscribes to the C.H.E.K theory could have an interesting time analyzing the numerous exercises and exercise systems. (For the interested reader, I have outlined how Swiss Ball training contributes to evaluation and improving functional movement in the video set *Advanced Swiss Ball Training for Rehabilitation*[12]).

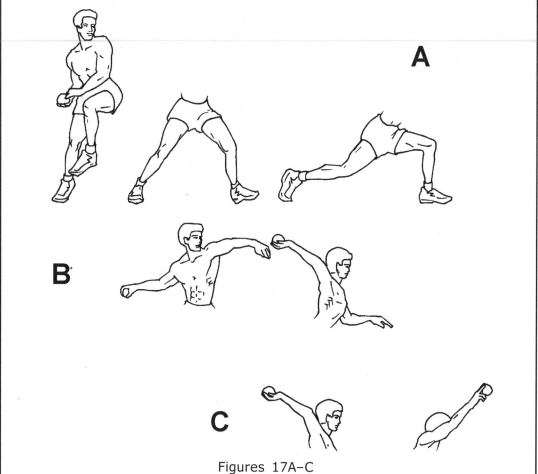

Figures 17A–C

A. The feet being the only point of contact with the ground necessitates that the body produce a lunge pattern to accelerate the torso.
B. Accelerating the torso into a twist pattern serves to windup the abdominal musculature, taking full advantage of length/force relationships while accelerating the shoulder/arm complex.
C. The push pattern is now expressed on top of the lunge-twist as a final summation of forces rising up the body, culminating with an explosive release at the point of optimal integration. It should be noted that a disorder in any of the individual patterns expressed as a "throw" will result in reduced performance and may eventually manifest as injury, usually at the weakest point in the kinetic chain.

Case History

A professional baseball pitcher was referred to me for a shoulder-conditioning program after having surgery to correct anterior subluxation of his right glenohumeral joint (shoulder). The pitcher (MB) stated that he had been having problems with his shoulder that began roughly 2½ years prior. He mentioned that the conditioning program he had been using was unable to stabilize the joint, and the team doctors determined that surgery was necessary. After having surgery he was concerned the problem could re-occur, particularly since prior conditioning programs had not worked. Therefore, he sought my consultation.

During my *Primal Pattern* assessment, I chose to have him throw a baseball-sized medicine ball at a rebounder. He was instructed to throw the ball using his standard pitching wind-up. I immediately noticed that as he stepped across his right foot, he became unstable in the right knee and did not effectively rotate the pelvis around his femur, nor his trunk around his pelvis, which resulted in excessive action at the arm. This type of problem is often referred to as "the tail wagging the dog" (Figures 18A–C).

This observation triggered me to ask MB if he felt any pain or discomfort in his right foot, leg, pelvis or spine as he threw the ball. He stated that he had been suffering from a bad case of turf toe for some time now and it hurt to step across the mound when he pitched. Further questioning determined that his toe had begun giving him problems three years ago. His shoulder began to hurt approximately 2½ years ago!

Evaluation of his right foot found what is technically referred to as *hallux rigidus*; the big toe cannot extend to the necessary 60-90° for functional gait and throwing activities. This is critical to understand because to pitch a ball or throw any object with speed requires that the body accelerate the torso with a lunge, upon which trunk rotation and the push (medial shoulder rotation, elbow extension and wrist flexion) are superimposed. In MB's case, he could not effectively accelerate his trunk due to inhibition of the stabilizers and prime movers of his right leg, which destabilized his trunk; the only way he could accelerate the ball to high speed was to accentuate the action of the arm in the push pattern, which resulted in shoulder injury.

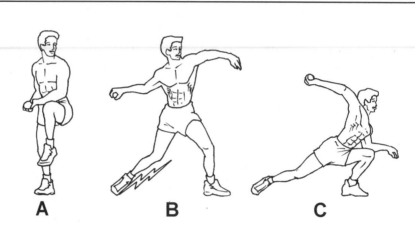

Figures 18A–C

The professional pitcher's hallux rigidus caused significant pain with dorsiflexion of the right great toe.

A. In an attempt to avoid dorsiflexion of the right great toe, he keeps his wind-up more vertical and reduces ankle plantar flexion (compare to Figure 17A).

B. Inability to utilize the right leg for force generation secondary to pain at the right great toe not only hinders wind-up of the torso, but the pain also produces inhibition of the torso musculature to minimize kinetic forces traveling back down the leg to the ground (compare to Figure 16).

C. Attempting to avoid dorsiflexion of the right great toe results in external rotation of the leg, stressing the medial collateral ligament of the knee, reducing force transfer from the ground and disrupting the timing of the pitch. To compensate for inability to use the leg and trunk properly, yet accelerate the ball to >90 MPH, he must excessively wind-up the shoulder and over-utilize the left leg.

The result of such a compensation pattern was shoulder instability that was treated surgically!

To further test my hypothesis, I placed three mats on the ground and rolled one into a makeshift mound for him to step across. He was then instructed to pitch the medicine ball at the rebounder again, using the same perceived effort. When he threw the medicine ball this time, it went so fast it came off the rebounder and almost tore the ceiling panels out of my gym! Needless to say, MB was shocked at what had just happened! I explained to MB that by making a mound from soft rubber material, he was able to move across his leg without excessive jamming of the great toe joint (first MTP), therefore the leg was not reflexively inhibited. This allowed him to effectively anchor his leg, transferring force upward from the ground while simultaneously allowing proper sequencing and summation of forces from the leg to the trunk, arm and finally into the hand and thus into the ball for release. It was suggested that MB consult a podiatrist for a "rocker shoe," which would allow weight transfer with minimal stress on the painful, degenerate great toe joint.

The important point to derive from this case history is that when looking at any compound movement pattern, it is critical to realize that any dysfunctional *Primal Pattern* movement will express itself throughout the entire kinetic chain. The magnitude of that expression will be proportional to that particular pattern's contribution to the overall compound movement pattern. In this case, the lunge is critical to the compound pattern we know as the throw pattern. The lunge dysfunction was compensated for by the shoulder, leading to shoulder injury.

For more information on how to prescribe exercises based on the *Primal Pattern* system, consult Paul Chek's *Advanced Program Design* Correspondence Course.[11]

4. OPEN- vs. CLOSED- CHAIN EXERCISE SELECTION

Although the concept of open- and closed-chain movements is under scrutiny by several elite physical therapists and conditioning specialists, I find the principles to be very useful. Originally popularized in medical literature by Arthur

C. Steindler, an open-chain movement can be broken down to indicate a movement in which you, the exerciser, can overcome the object you are applying force to. It may also be considered a movement in which the distal segment is free to move.[13] A closed-chain is said to exist if you cannot overcome the object your body is pushing against, or a movement in which the distal segment is fixed. A simple example to illustrate the principles of open- and closed-chain movements can be seen when comparing the lat pull-down exercise (open-chain) to the chin-up (closed-chain). No matter how hard you pull on a chin-up bar, you are not going to pull it out of a squat cage, but you will eventually pull your body past the bar, since the chain is closed and you have applied adequate force to lift your own body weight. The lat pull-down, on the other hand, will be an open-chain exercise until such time that you increase the load to the point at which you can no longer open the chain. At that point, you will be doing a chin-up from the lat pull-down bar!

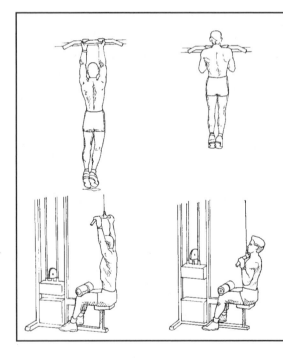

Figure 19
During the open-chain lat pull-down, the distal segment is free to move. During the closed-chain chin-up, the distal segment is fixed. Careful observation of open- vs. closed-chain exercises with similar movement structures, such as seen here, will demonstrate that the sequencing of movements in open- vs. closed-chain exercises are 180° out of phase with each other, as are the osteokinematics (bone movements).

Now, regardless of what the various "industry experts" say about open- and closed-chain not being relevant, I beleive that anyone who has done any athletic training for sports such as rock climbing, gymnastics or even for military competitions will soon tell you that the lat pull-down exercise does very little to improve chin-up performance. In fact, if you look at the arthrokinematics of the two movements, you will see that during the chin-up, the body must pull itself past a fixed hand, while during the lat pull-down the load and arms must be pulled toward and across a fixed torso and rib cage. Therefore, it is safe to say the recruitment patterns generated by the nervous system in each exercise are 180° out of phase with each other!

To give you an example of how one movement can be performed 180° out of phase with another and yield little result, consider an old-fashioned record player. If the record player turns clockwise at the correct speed, it produces music, but if it turns counterclockwise at the same speed, it makes noise! Both the lat pull-down and the chin-up exercises can produce big muscles, but are the big muscles under optimal neurological command to perform the movement at task?

Application: To make the most of the time spent training with any client or patient, try to choose exercises that resemble the environment of application with regard to open- and closed-chain principles.

5. FUNCTIONAL EXERCISE IMPROVES RELEVANT BIOMOTOR ABILITIES

Biomotor can be broken down into its component parts to give its full meaning: bio = life, and motor = movement. Tudor Bompa describes the importance of biomotor abilities in his book *Theory and Methodology of Strength Training.*[14] Biomotor abilities consist of such qualities as those listed in Table 3.

• Agility	• Endurance
• Balance	• Flexibility
• Coordination	• Power
• Strength and its components such as start, explosive and finish strength	

Table 3

Understanding the concept of biomotor abilities is important when determining how functional an exercise is. Most functional exercises, as dictated by the guidelines presented here, address multiple biomotor abilities, but the focus may be on one specific biomotor ability. For example, the multidirectional lunge exercise (Figure 20), regardless of acute exercise variable selection, will improve, or at least serve to maintain, some level of balance, coordination, flexibility and agility. By manipulation of acute exercise variables you can also include power, strength or endurance.

If you simply compare the multidirectional lunge, a functional exercise, to a Smith machine split squat (the only machine-based exercise that has any real relationship from a movement perspective), you will see that the only variables remaining are flexibility and whatever force-generating quality selected via acute exercise variables. By using the machine for stabilization, one loses the ability to improve balance, agility and coordination beyond the intermuscular coordination that is a given for any compound exercise. Even intermuscular coordination demands are decreased when stabilized by a machine.

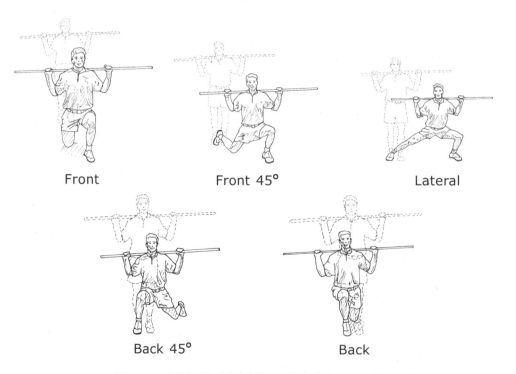

Front   Front 45°   Lateral

Back 45°   Back

Figures 20A–E: Multidirectional Lunge Exercise

Application: To determine how functional any exercise is with regard to biomotor ability and biomotor ability development, simply ask yourself these questions.

1. Does the exercise I am about to use improve the biomotor abilities the client needs to improve for the specific goals of their program and the needs of their body?

2. Am I giving the client an exercise that is too simple, or one that *under-challenges* their nervous system?

3. Is the goal of the exercise neuromuscular-isolation or neuromuscular-integration? (Neuromuscular-isolation exercises are often best performed on machines or with the support of benches and props, such as preacher benches, while a neuromuscular-integration exercise is usually best performed at the most demanding level possible without disrupting the motor learning process.)

4. Does this exercise have the optimal biomotor profile for developing my client's skill level and movement patterns? The tendency most exercise and rehabilitation professionals have is to go to either extreme: The exercises are either far too simplistic (machine) or far too complex (Pro-Fitter lateral slides catching a medicine ball).

Choosing the exercise that best addresses the biomotor requirements of your client's environment and one that suits their motor skills development can only serve to speed the rate at which they achieve their conditioning or rehabilitation goals!

6. ISOLATE, THEN INTEGRATE!

In the video correspondence course *Scientific Back Training*, I speak of the rule I developed: "If you are going to isolate, you must then integrate."[19] As the trainer of the U.S.

Army Boxing Team, I saw many examples of what happens to good athletes who spend too much time on machines or isolation exercises.

Movement for any work or sports environment, regardless of the exact type, requires that we develop movement, or motor skills. Isolation exercises, as the name implies, *isolate.* Improving movement skill can only be accomplished by integration. Do not take this to mean there is no place for isolation exercises. For example, if someone has had a C4/5 disc bulge and developed atrophy of the deltoid and rotator cuff musculature as a result, an isolation exercise could be prescribed to stimulate hypertrophy as quickly and effectively as possible. However, integrating these muscles and joints with the rest of the body is paramount in the rehabilitation process.

Application: Using the above example of atrophy of the C5 innervated musculature of the shoulder, we would have to develop the infraspinatus and deltoids of the involved shoulder. To do this, we would first perform isolation exercises for the rotator cuff. If the cuff was not strong enough to handle dynamic exercise of the deltoid, one might assess to see if isometric exercises were safe. If not, then we would first rehabilitate the rotator cuff to sufficient levels of function to accommodate deltoid exercises.

A classic example of progression for this case would be as follows.

1. Isolation training for the external shoulder rotators
2. Integration for the external shoulder rotators
3. Isolation training for the deltoid
    - Isometric and/or super slow tempo training first
    - Dynamic training for the shoulder with a fully functional rotator cuff
4. Integration training for the deltoid group
    - Pushing
    - Pulling
    - Combined patterns training

10 TIPS FOR OPTIMAL MOTOR LEARNING

1. IDENTIFY YOUR CLIENT'S LEARNING STYLE

Learning experts have identified seven types of intelligences, all of which directly influence the way we most effectively learn.[15] These are verbal/linguistic, logical/mathematical, visual/spatial, intrapersonal, interpersonal, musical and physical/kinesthetic. It is estimated that about 95% of all the information we learn in school comes prepackaged in a verbal/linguistic or logical/mathematical form, which is fantastic for those naturally endowed with one or both of those learning styles.[15] It is also the reason why highly kinesthetic individuals find themselves visiting the principal more frequently. I should know, I was one of those kids!

To identify your client's most effective learning style or intelligence, simply ask them, "Do you learn best by having things explained to you, physically doing things, watching before doing, or by reading a diagram or description and then attempting the task at hand?" The student will typically prefer one specific style but may prefer a combination of learning styles, which will likely match their intelligence profile.

Once you have learned which way they most effectively learn, use that knowledge to teach them how to move. In fact, if you think of clients you have worked with in the past, clients that you thought were "motor morons," chances are very good that you were teaching them with a *teaching style* that did not match their *learning style.*

PREPARE THE ENVIRONMENT FOR LEARNING

When teaching motor skills or "movement," it is critical to prepare the environment to facilitate the learning process. Environmental factors that often affect learning are:

Space. If there is inadequate space to perform the movement task at hand, it is likely to detract from the learning process. For example, I have had to try to teach lunging exercises in various gyms around the world, many of which were so cluttered with exercise machines that it was impossible to find sufficient space to perform a lunge exercise. Dodging machines adds an unwanted element of distraction to the learning process.

Cleanliness. Another very important aspect to consider when teaching movement is cleanliness. Just as it can be cumbersome to teach movement skills in a gym full of body-building machines, trying to teach lunging, pushing, pulling, twisting and most other movements can be both challenging and dangerous if the floor is not clean. This is particularly true in cases where an apparatus such as the Swiss Ball must be used to either ascend the exercise (make it harder) or descend the exercise (make it easier). The learning environment should not have a foul smell either. As most of you are aware, many gyms smell of old sweat, sometimes mold, dust and other unpleasant odors! Such smells are not only distracting, but can trigger allergic responses in your client, which often include "mental fog" as a physiological response. This does not aid the learning experience.

Lighting. It is not uncommon to enter a gym that is poorly illuminated. When the lighting is poor it makes it very hard to see joint structures, soft tissue and bony landmarks and overall movement characteristics. When lighting is poor, concentration is also poor. Because cortisol is an activating hormone and cortisol rhythm follows the sun (higher levels in the body in the morning, decreasing as the sun goes down) (16), attempting to teach someone in an environment where their brain thinks it is bedtime is not favorable.

Music. Today there are a huge number of gyms playing everything from grunge and acid rock to rap and hip-hop music. For nearly everyone, such music is not conducive to learning. In fact, it is not conducive to exercise! A study conducted at Louisiana State University found that listening to hard-driving rock music increased heart rates and lowered the quality of workouts in a group of 24 young adults.[17] John Diamond, M.D., found that "weakening beats," from groups such as The Doors, Janis Joplin, Queen, Alice Cooper, and Led Zeppelin (among others) caused a loss of symmetry between the left and right cerebral hemispheres, inducing subtle perceptual difficulties and a host of other early manifestations of stress.[18] Some of the changes Diamond found included decreased performance in school, hyperactivity, restlessness, decreased work output, increased errors, decreased decision-making capacity and a feeling that things just aren't right. Interestingly, he found that listening to The Beatles never produced such negative effects.[18]

Although there are numerous studies available on the effects of music on learning and the body, it is generally understood that classical music from the Baroque time period facilitates learning, jazz neither facilitates nor inhibits learning in most cases, and most rock music disrupts learning. Therefore, to create an environment that facilitates teaching your client how to move correctly, classical music, jazz, and if you must, the Beatles, may be your best choices.

2. ABILITY QUALIFICATION

When teaching your client a particular movement, it is imperative that you qualify their *ability* to perform that given movement. If you are trying to teach a client to perform a lunge, and they have a degenerative hip joint that will only extend to 5°, they will have trouble performing the lunge, no matter how good your instructional skills are. This is a very common problem in the sport of golf today. The majority of golfers are above 35 years of age and many have *ability limitations,* yet instructors routinely try to get such people to swing the club like Tiger Woods. To teach a movement without first qualifying the client's ability or orthopedic capacity to perform the movement only results in compensation patterns and increases the chances of injury and/or re-injury. An example of a comparative range of motion assessment is well described in *Scientific Back Training.*[9]

3. AVOID PAIN!

When teaching any movement pattern, it is CRITICAL to avoid pain. According to Vladimir Janda, pain is a more powerful reprogramming stimulus than any therapeutic agent known to man![19] Janda also stated that is it very important to avoid any deeply ingrained motor pattern when pain is present.[19] For example, when treating an injured runner with knee pain, it is detrimental to attempt correcting gait mechanics if there is any appreciation of pain during the gait cycle. Pain not only causes inhibition in the nervous system and weakens any muscle crossing the weight-bearing joints, but it also immediately results in production of compensatory movement patterns. These are unlikely to be as efficient and effective as the original pattern (Figures 18A–C and associated case history).

4. RANDOM vs. BLOCK PRACTICE

Random training is exposure to a task or lesson at random. In block training, specific blocks of time are set aside for the purpose of accomplishing a given task or to learn a skill. An example given by Schmidt of random vs. block training is learning to use a mathematical formula.[10] Block training suggests you perform equation after equation using the same formula, while random training dictates that you will be exposed to the equation at random. In a random training format, you would have to go through the thought process of how to apply the formula each time you applied it, while with block training you simply apply the same thought process over and over again.

Current literature on motor learning suggests that for long-term retention of a skill, random exposures provide the best results. Block training often provides better results initially, but random exposure appears to produce better long-term outcomes because each time you are exposed to a task at random, your brain is tasked with problem-solving, ultimately improving function.[10,20,21]

The practitioner may capitalize on this information when working to develop new motor skills by scheduling enough blocks of training to allow initial development of a new skill. After the skill is learned adequately, the practitioner may then progress learning by switching from one skill to another at *random.* An example of the difference is commonly seen in golf. Many people opt for *block practice* at the driving range, hitting 100–300 balls per *block* of training. When the player goes to the golf course, he/she must select the appropriate motor pattern or skill at random, as dictated by the game.

5. COGNITIVE ASSOCIATION

Cognitive association, or the thought process associated with any motor task, may have a tremendous influence upon outcome. This is very important to remember when testing an individual's motor skills, or you may mistakenly

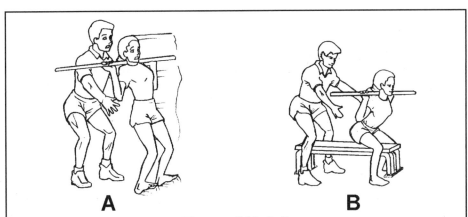

A   B

Figures 21A & B

A. When asked to "squat," the person with no cognitive association with the term or command "squat" often can't organize an effective motor response. In this situation, clients/patients frequently fall backward or freeze. **B.** By asking the same client/patient to "lower yourself to the bench as though to sit, but stop just short," the brain produces a movement the therapist/trainer observes as a squat because of the commonality in relative timing (generalized motor program). This example serves to show that there is a cognitive relationship between the command given and the motor program selected in the brain.

underestimate the client's motor capacity. A common example I have seen numerous times in the clinic occurs while testing the squat movement pattern.

If you take a client into the clinic or gym and send them to the squat rack to squat, or simply ask them to demonstrate a squat, many of them will either tell you, "I don't know how" or they will attempt a squat and may fall over backward (Figure 21A)! After falling over backward into the arms of an assistant or the therapist, I have asked the client what they were thinking when that happened. They stated "I don't know, it just happened. I guess I don't know how to squat!"

Now, having observed the same clients getting into and out of chairs in the waiting area, I can assure you, *they do know how to squat.* With this knowledge, I repeat the test again, but this time I change the *cognitive association* by simply asking them to sit down on the weightlifting bench as though they were sitting in a chair. Presto, they squat (Figure 21B)! The client will often make a comment such as, "Oh, is that what you wanted? Why didn't you just ask?" This provides strong evidence that the brain stores the movement pattern with cognitive association or connection to the task most associated with the use of that particular movement pattern.

Another example can be seen in the Park Ranger, who when asked to lunge has a vague idea of what is expected (Figure 22A). When asking the same Park Ranger to step forward as though stepping over a fallen tree in the forest, he can produce a lunge without hesitation (Figure 22B).

To capitalize on this information, you must always ask your client what type of work and sports activities they have performed in the past and which activities they currently take part in. This knowledge will serve to guide you toward pre-framing them, or facilitating the selection of the movement pattern stored in their sensory-motor system that most closely resembles the pattern you desire to assess.

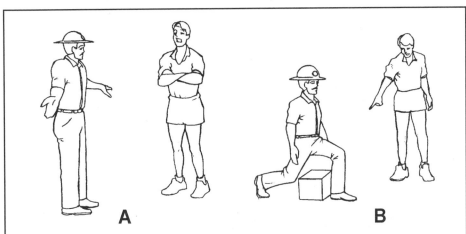

Figures 22A & B

A. The therapist/trainer trying to assess movement skill in a Park Ranger with no background in guided exercise has no motor association with the command "Lunge, please." B. When a box is placed on the ground and the Park Ranger is asked to demonstrate how he would cross a log laying across a trail he was traveling, he clearly demonstrates that the lunge pattern was not stored in his brain under the command "lunge" but was easily retrieved with the command "step across the log."

6. TEACHING MOVEMENT IN CHUNKS

Motor learning research shows that the body learns to move, or develops motor programs, in *chunks*. In motor learning, *chunking* is defined as "the combining of individual elements in memory into larger units."[22] In Figures 17A–C, the baseball pitch, or throw pattern, has been broken down into the three most likely chunks: *the lunge, the twist and the push.*

As described by Schmidt and Lee, when learning a motor program, the motor program is developed in *chunks* that are stored in short-term memory.[22] As mastery is developed over each given chunk, it will be the basis of what often becomes a larger motor program. As each chunk is learned, the brain begins to tie the chunks together, provided they can be accessed by the same cognitive command. For example, using the breakdown of the throw pattern demonstrated in Figures 17A–C, it is possible to see what could be considered three chunks having been tied together by the brain to become one large, complex motor program. The baseball player, after adequate training, could now access this information by simply thinking "pitch," or "throw the ball."

Chunking can be used as an effective teaching technique by breaking movements down into their distinctive parts. Using the Single-Arm Cable Push exercise as an example (Figures 23A–C), the obvious first step to teach is the weight shift, or proper use of the legs (Figure 23A). This is followed by learning how to use the trunk on top of the legs to twist and summate trunk forces with leg forces (Figure 23B). Finally the client is taught when to most effectively integrate the *push* for optimal summation of leg-trunk forces and maximal efficiency of the shoulder (Figure 23C).[23] Once learned as separate chunks, the complete movement is stored in long-term memory and can be recalled as a single motor program.

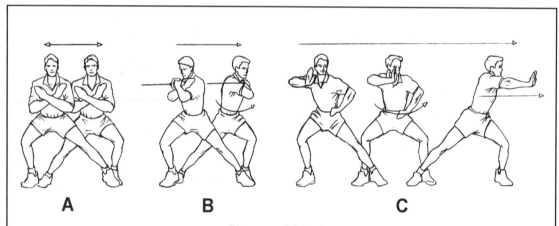

Figures 23A–C

A. First the weight shift, which has similar timing to the lunge pattern, is taught.

B. Once the weight shift/lunge is mastered, the twist pattern is superimposed upon it.

C. The push pattern, which is ultimately a combination of the lunge and twist with the push superimposed, is taught after mastering the previously demonstrated *chunks,* or *smaller motor programs.* Teaching movement in this manner is easy for the instructor to do, easy for the client to learn, and ultimately results in reduced incidence of injury.

7. MOVEMENT SPEED

When teaching movement, there is an optimal movement speed for both learning movements and for assessing movements.[23]

In general, when teaching strength movements, such as the squat, bent-over row, dead lift or bench press, *slow* tempos of execution are most effective. At the C.H.E.K Institute we consider a *slow tempo* to be a 1-2-3 count. Teaching the dead lift from the rack on a *slow* tempo would require that your student lower the bar for a count of 1-2-3 and raise the bar for a count of 1-2-3.

The slower tempo gives the student a chance to use feedback from their own body while learning to control the load. It also gives the teacher a chance to see what is happening and where any movement fault may originate from. Using a slow tempo while teaching a strength-training movement is also helpful because if the student loses control of the load, the teacher has a chance to spot them, guiding their movements for better motor learning.

When teaching body-weight movements such as lunging, box step-ups or exercises that require a high degree of balance (such as the snatch lift), a moderate tempo or slightly faster movement is best. As you can imagine from your experience with these types of exercises, if moving too slowly while balancing on one leg, or trying to accelerate a load as in the snatch, a lack of balance or motor deficiency will be magnified. This would only serve to teach poor movement.

When assessing your client's movement skills, it is often necessary to slow the movement down so you can see what is happening. For example, with a box step-up exercise you can simply ask the client to step up or down more slowly so you can observe how they use their body. While looking at a snatch, clean and jerk, or power clean, it is not practical or realistic to ask someone to slow down too much because it disrupts the timing of the movement; in this case it is much better to use video analysis so you can control the speed of the tape for observational purposes.

8. FEEDBACK, THE BREAKFAST OF CHAMPIONS!

Have you ever been working out in the gym and had a friend say, "Did you know your back was rounding," or "Do you realize you are raising the bar faster on the right than the left?" At the time you received that *feedback,* you probably thought, "Was I really doing that?" or "I wonder how long that's been happening?" The point is, EVEN THE VERY BEST TEACHERS, THERAPISTS AND ATHLETES CAN BENEFIT FROM FEEDBACK.

Feedback is commonly classified into *intrinsic feedback, extrinsic feedback* and *knowledge of results*:[10]

INTRINSIC vs. EXTRINSIC FEEDBACK

Intrinsic feedback is feedback you can obtain using your own senses. For example, when driving a golf ball, you can often tell if your shot will be good before you even hit the ball because you can sense your body and club position as well as speed through your proprioceptive system. Once ball contact is made, you can use your own eyesight to assess whether what you felt matches what actually happened. In otherwords, did the ball fly straight and as far as you *felt* it would?

Extrinsic feedback enhances the feedback you received from your intrinsic sources. It is information that you could not obtain yourself and often comes from a coach, therapist, timing device or video camera. Extrinsic feedback provides *knowledge of results.* According to Schmidt, research shows that when the learner cannot detect his/her own errors, without *knowledge of results,* learning does not take place.[10, 22]

To effectively use intrinsic and extrinsic feedback and to skillfully apply knowledge of results, consider the following tips.

✓   Ask the client for feedback. Whenever possible, ask your client what they *felt* during the movement you are teaching them. This allows them to become more tuned into their proprioceptive systems, ultimately elevating their sense of body awareness. This is particularly important in sports such as football, wrestling and weightlifting and in jobs such as heavy construction or farming where athletes and workers must handle heavy loads. If your client is unaware of their body position under load, their chance of injury is much greater.

✓ Do not give extrinsic feedback too soon. It is important not to give extrinsic feedback until you have had a chance to determine your client's level of kinesthetic awareness with regard to their body sense or positional sense. This is important, particularly for those who have endured a past injury or have had limited exposure to movement stimuli. These clients often have *sensory-motor amnesia,* which implies the body is unable to sense where it is in space and therefore cannot organize an appropriate motor response. Asking the client, "What do you feel you could have improved during that lunge?" for example, makes them become aware of their intrinsic information sources.

If your client is unable to give you adequate feedback with regard to what they *felt during the exercise,* then you must foster learning by giving them *extrinsic feedback,* or *knowledge of results.* It is at this time that you will aid the learning process by telling them, "Your back leg was too straight and your upper back was rounded." If upon receiving this information they still cannot make the correction, you will most likely have to use other sources of extrinsic feedback, such as video or palpation. By providing palpatory cues, the client not only has an immediate source of extrinsic feedback, they also have heightened intrinsic feedback, which often significantly reduces learning time.

✓ Focus on the major faults. When providing extrinsic feedback, always focus on the *primary issue* first. You don't want to induce paralysis by analysis! If you tell your client seven things they did wrong with the movement or exercise they just performed, they are likely to be overwhelmed by the information and have a hard time integrating even one piece of it into the next movement. Look for the *single greatest movement fault,* particularly a *catalyst fault,* or one that affects several other factors. By correcting the biggest fault, especially if it is a catalyst fault, you will not overload your client's brain and may see rapid improvements in their movement skill!

✓ Use props. When your client has a hard time correcting body position or movement, even after soliciting intrinsic feedback and offering extrinsic feedback, it is often beneficial to use props. One of my favorite props for developing enhanced motor skill is athletic tape. For example, in patients who cannot sense where their lumbar spine is during a *Primal Pattern* movement, I stand them upright and tape their lumbar spine in a neutral position by running tape on either side of the spine from T12 to S2. This way every time they lose their lumbar position they have enhanced proprioceptive input. The tape often serves to enhance their position sense, resulting in a better opportunity to give more positive extrinsic feedback, and thus speed the learning process.

9. TRAIN, DON'T DRAIN!

The old "no pain, no gain" approach to exercise that permeated training environments such as the military, football and bodybuilding gyms, unfortunately continues to influence the rehabilitative and professional exercise community. This is a viewpoint that is counterproductive and must be modified if your clients are to see lasting results.

To truly improve movement skill and performance in any client, we must adhere to a few basic principles of motor learning and physiology. For example, we must stop thinking of time spent in the gym as a "*workout.*" The word "work" is something that immediately turns off many of the people we see as clients. Some people do not like to exert themselves, and many people do not cherish the thought of sweating! The word "out" when tacked on to the word "work" implies working until the end, or until you are literally "out" like a car out of gas! This form of cognitive association worked well in a sport like football where the most common expression of motor skill is exploding off the line and hitting your opponent hard enough to induce a state of semiconsciousness, much like a bird flying into a window! But this is not the best choice of words for most people!

"Working out" also serves to describe what is done in bodybuilding to build muscle mass. You go to the gym, and using machines and isolation exercises, you work the muscle into oblivion, breaking down as much protein as possible, knowing full well that the body will respond with a rebound response that results in increased muscle mass over time. Now let's be honest here – if you had to rate bodybuilding exercises for their average level of motor complexity on a scale of 10, 10 being very complex, then a score of 1–4 would be fair. With that in mind, why in the world would we ever want to let such tactics, exercises and primitive principles enter into the world of rehabilitation and professional exercise instruction? *It constantly amazes me!*

Teaching movement is teaching skill . . . it's that simple. Functional exercise requires movement skills ranging all the way to 10 out of 10 on the complexity scale. Therefore, we should look more closely at what it takes to build good motor programs.

TRAIN THE MOVEMENT, NOT THE MUSCLE

The body knows nothing of muscles, only of movement.[24] During the constant adaptive changes that must take place in order to preserve our equilibrium while moving, the body is constantly activating an array of muscles in patterns of coordination, in which muscles lose their identity.[24] When we train *movements,* we train hundreds of muscles at once. To teach *functional movement* requires meeting all components of functional movement or functional exercise described earlier in this chapter.

When you have hundreds of muscles on the job, you have a massive increase in demand for neurological energy and metabolic resources. The central and peripheral nervous systems have a finite amount of energy available at any given time and are subject to fatigue. This is critical when you consider that the brain is inefficient, consuming some 80% of available blood sugar. Brain fuel consumption will rise during such activities as learning a new movement or taking a test. I am sure you have all had the experience of taking a long test and walking out afterward feeling fatigued.

The nervous system is subject to greater levels of fatigue while:

1. in a learning state
2. performing exercises that require activation of a massive muscle population
3. requiring minimal base of support and/or high levels of motor complexity.

Knowing this, it becomes evident that carefully scheduled rest periods are critical to the overall quality of learning and the learning experience. Frank Wildman, Ph.D., a Feldenkrais teacher, tells his class that Feldenkrais himself suggested that no one should ever work at learning a new exercise for longer than two minutes at a time, or mental fatigue from the learning process would impede the quality of learning.

What I am suggesting here is that we step away from the *workout* model and step into a *training* model. This model focuses on the *quality of movement learned* and the understanding that the body is a biocellular computer, a programmable sensory-motor system. But like any computer, it is only capable of outputting movements of a quality directly proportional to the quality of the motor inputs we have programmed into it!

I am not suggesting that we stay away from *strength-training,* I am merely suggesting that we "*train,* and not *drain*"the body while in the developmental stages. After your client has demonstrated proficiency with the relevant motor patterns, you can begin strength training, building upon a sound neuromechanical and sensory-motor foundation. The result can only be a stronger client with less chance of injury!

10. PERFECT PRACTICE, MAKES PERFECT!

Tony Robbins and other self-help gurus can be heard saying, "Repetition is the mother of skill." When it comes to motor learning and teaching movement, repetition is the mother of skill, *provided there is skill in the repetitions!*

Ultimately, we are trying to progress each client through the three stages of learning:[10,20,22, 26]

1. the verbal cognitive stage (associated with talking to yourself and thinking it through)
2. the motor stage (the assembled program is now being refined)
3. the autonomous stage (running the motor program with the mind free to be elsewhere).

A good estimate is that it may take 300 repetitions to get to the stage of automaticity.[10] This is not very many repetitions in most gym or practice situations, particularly when you consider that it is common for an aspiring golfer to go to the driving range and hit 100–300 balls in one afternoon, or that a Little Leaguer practicing his pitching with Dad may easily throw over 100 pitches in one outing!

Now, let us consider the Law of Facilitation, which states, "When an impulse has passed once through a certain set of neurons to the exclusion of others, it will tend to take the same course on a future occasion, and each time it traverses this path the resistance in the path will be smaller."[25] What this means in English is that every time you allow your client to perform a repetition of an exercise or movement incorrectly, it becomes *easier and easier for them to do it incorrectly and harder and harder for them to do it correctly!*

When teaching or maintaining any motor skill, it is critical to remember that the most powerful stimuli for programming the nervous system are *pain* and *emotion.* At the onset of central and peripheral nervous system fatigue, performance begins to dwindle, often resulting in frustration and elevated emotional states, particularly after having performed well. Because the nervous system responds to the *greatest stimuli,* one must consider how many attempts were optimal and how many were sub-optimal? If your response is greater than 50% suboptimal and you become emotional about it, experience pain, or both, you are progressively developing *faulty motor programs* (Figures 24A–C)! This fact should not be taken lightly, considering clinical experience dictates that it may take between 3,000 and 5,500 repetitions to override a faulty motor program with a new motor program. This is exactly why it is said that you can't teach an old dog new tricks!

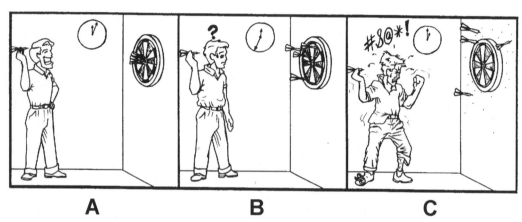

A   **B**   **C**

Figures 24A-C

Today in rehabilitation, professional exercise and sports training alike, there is a great propensity to *over-train,* resulting in poor sensory-motor programming secondary to nervous system fatigue.

A. Initially, the aspiring performer often performs well. This level of performance will have a time window that varies from person-to-person.

B. When pushed past the *window of optimal performance and motor learning,* performance begins to drop, which is often stressful to the performer.

C. With dogmatic determination and progressive central nervous system fatigue, fine motor control diminishes, performance dwindles and negative emotional states begin to take front stage! It is critical to remember *the nervous system is most easily and effectively programmed in the presence of pain and emotion.* The greatest stimulus ultimately dictates what is learned. What do you think is being learned here?

To capitalize on this valuable, clinically tried and tested information, simply focus on developing *quality of movement first.* Do not worry about how much your client is lifting or what the "Jones'" are doing! Once you have programmed the sensory-motor system with *optimal* movement skills, then begin developing improved strength, and finally improve power output or the speed at which the movement pattern can be produced under load if necessary.

CONCLUSION

This has been a brief summary of what the C.H.E.K Institute uses for guidelines to teach functional movement and to determine the validity of an exercise as "functional." As you can see, virtually every exercise in the world can become functional at some point in a spectrum of rehabilitation. Part of the art, science and skill of being a superior conditioning or rehabilitation professional is knowing when to progress the client so that the maximum opportunity for learning and development are not missed. Let us all move into the new Millennium with an elevated consciousness about movement. Let us all head to the gym and "*train, not drain!*"

REFERENCES

1. Abreu, B. C. Physical Disabilities Manual. New York, NY: Raven Press, 1981.

2. Barnes, M., Crutchfield, C., & Cummings, G. Orthopedic Physical Therapy Series. Atlanta, GA: Stokesville Publishing Co., 1985.

3. Hypes, B. Facilitating Development and Sensorimotor Function. PDP Press, 1991.

4. Janda, V., Function of Muscles and Musculoskeletal Pain Syndromes – A Lab Course. San Diego, CA, April 1999.

5. Chek, P. The Golf Biomechanic's Manual. San Diego, CA: A C.H.E.K Institute publication, 1999.

6. Andersson, Gunnar, & Chaffin, D.B., Occupational Biomechanics. 2nd Edition. New York, NY: John Wiley & Sons, Inc., 1990.

7. Guyton, Arthur, Textbook of Medical Physiology. Philadelphia, PA: W.B. Saunders Company, 1986.

8. Richardson, C. et al. Therapeutic Exercise for Spinal Segmental Stabilization in Low Back Pain. Edinburgh: Churchill Livingstone, 1999.

9. Chek, P. Scientific Back Training, correspondence course and videocassette series. San Diego, CA: A C.H.E.K Institute publication and production, 1993.

10. Schmidt, R.H. Motor Learning and Performance. Champaign, IL: Human Kinetics, 1991.

11. Chek, P. Advanced Program Design, correspondence course and video cassette series. San Diego, CA: A C.H.E.K Institute publication and production, 1998.

12. Chek, P. Advanced Swiss Ball Training for Rehabilitation, video cassette series. San Diego, CA: A C.H.E.K Institute production, 2000.

13. Steindler, Arthur. Kinesiology of the Human Body. Springfield, IL: Charles C. Thomas, 1964.

14. Bompa, Tudor. <u>Theory & Methodology of Training.</u> Dubuque, IA: Kendall/Hunt Publishing Company, 1983.

15. Lazear David. <u>Seven Ways of Teaching (2nd Ed.) – The Artistry of Teaching with Multiple Intelligences</u>. Hawker Brownlow Education, Australia, 1991.

16. Timmins, Bill, Naturopathic Physician. Personal Communication. San Diego, CA, 1999.

17. Campbell, Don, <u>The Mozart Effect</u>. New York, NY: Avon Books, 1997.

18. Diamond, John, <u>Your Body Doesn't Lie.</u> New York, NY: Warner Books, 1979.

19. Janda, Vladimir. "Function of Muscles and Musculoskeletal Pain Syndromes." San Diego, CA, April 1999.

20. Schmidt, R. A. <u>Motor Learning and Performance Instructor's Guide</u>. Champaign, IL: Human Kinetics, 1992.

21. Magill, R.A. <u>Motor Learning – Concepts and Applications</u>. 3rd Edition. Dubuque, IA: Wm. C. Brown Publishers, College Division, 1989.

22. Schmidt, R.A., Lee, T.D. <u>Motor Control and Learning – A Behavioral Emphasis</u> 3rd edition. Champaign, IL: Human Kinetics Publishers, 1999.

23. Chek, P. <u>Corrective High-performance Exercise Kinesiology – Level II Internship Course Manual</u>. San Diego, CA: A C.H.E.K Institute publication, 1995.

24. Bobath, K. "A Neurophysiological Basis for the Treatment of Cerebral Palsy." <u>Clinics in Developmental Medicine</u> No. 75. 2nd. Ed. of CDM 23. The Motor Deficit in Patients with Cerebral Palsy, Spactics International Medical Publications, 1980, London, William Heinemann Medical Books Ltd. Philadelphia: J.B. Lippincott Co.

25. <u>27th Ed. Dorland's Illustrated Medical Dictionary</u>. p. 900. Philadelphia, PA: W.B. Saunders Co., 1985.

26. Schmidt, R.A. and Wrisberg, C.A. <u>Motor Learning and Performance</u> 2nd Edition. Champaign, IL: Human Kinetics, 2000.

Index

A

ability 19, 34
agility 29, 30
ankle 26
athletic tape 44
autonomous stage 47
axis of rotation 13, 14, 15

B

balance 11, 29, 30, 41
base conditioning 18
baseball 40
    pitcher 25
bench press 16, 17, 41
bent-over row 9, 10, 41
biomotor ability 6, 29–31
block training 36
body sense 43

C

cable push exercise 17, 18, 40
center of gravity 6, 10–12, 18
chin-up 28, 29
chunking 39, 40
closed-chain 6, 27, 28
cognitive association 37, 38, 44
coordination 29, 30
core muscles 17, 24, 25
cortisol 34

D

dance 18
dead lift 15, 41
deltoid 32
disc bulge 32

E

endurance 29, 30
extension moment 12

F

faulty motor programs 48
feedback 41
    extrinsic 42, 43, 45
    intrinsic 42
Feldenkrais 46
flexibility 29, 30
flexion moment 12, 13
football 16, 43, 44
force generation 15, 26, 30
functional
    movement (exercise) 5, 6,
    11, 18, 21, 23, 29–31, 45
    strength 15

G

generalized motor program 19, 37
golf 42
Golgi tendon 16

H

hallux rigidus 25, 26
heart rate 34
hockey 11

I

integration 6, 32
    neuromuscular 18, 31
intermuscular coordination 30
isolation 6, 18, 19, 32, 45
    neuromuscular 31

J

Janda 8, 32
joint
    degeneration 14
    instability 13
    stabilizers 14

C.H.E.K Institute International Distributors

Canada
Fitter International
4515 1st St. SE
Calgary, AB T2G 2L2 Canada
1.800.FITTER1 or 403.243.6830
fax: 403.229.1230
fitter.international@home.com
www.fitter1.com

South Pacific
Highest Quality Health & Fitness
75 Sunrise Ave.
Murrays Bay, NSC New Zealand
1.800.552.8789 (Australia)
0.800.552.8789 (NZ)
+64.9.478.2111
fax: +64.9.478.9111
info@hqh.com
www.hqh.com

Europe
Paul Chek Seminars UK
18 St. Lawrence Mews
Sovereign Harbour North
Eastbourne, East Sussex, BN23 5QD
United Kingdom
0845.601.4279 (UK)
+44.1323.471.693
fax: +44.1323.471.069
alex@paulchekseminarsuk.com

GET HOOKED ON KNOWLEDGE ...

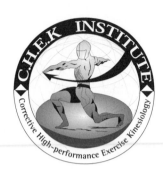

For more information on home study courses,
videos, books, equipment, certification
programs and consultations available from the
C.H.E.K Institute, contact us at:

609 S. Vulcan Ave. Ste. 101
Encinitas, CA 92024 USA
1.800.552.8789
760.632.6360
fax: 760.632.1037
ginfo@chekinstitute.com
www.chekinstitute.com

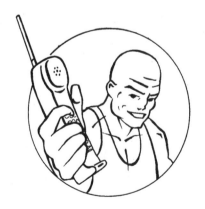